SWIMMING IN A TROPICAL SEA

A meditative story to massage your body
and relax your mind

BOOKS IN THE NATUREBODY™ SERIES

—

Walking in an Ancient Forest

Camping Under the Night Sky

Relaxing by a Waterfall

A Peaceful Winter Ski

Swimming in a Tropical Sea

A Healing Coastal Walk

Relaxing in the High Desert

A Spirited Mountain Hike

The complete
NatureBody™ Connection
program is available at

www.aquaterramassage.com

A NATUREBODY™ MASSAGE STORY

Swimming in a TROPICAL SEA

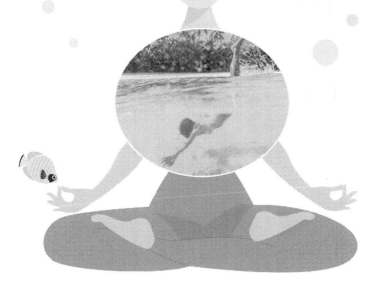

A meditative story to massage your body
and relax your mind

ERIK KRIPPNER *and* FAYE KRIPPNER

ISBN: 978-1-959772-05-7

Cover art provided by Envato Elements. Cover design by Faye Krippner and Erik Krippner.

Release Date for First Printed Edition 2023.

Media Inquiries: If you would like to contact the authors, please send an email to press@aquaterramassage.com.

Faye Krippner, B.A., LMT and Erik Krippner, B.S., LMT have been licensed by the Oregon Board of Massage Therapy since 2003. Oregon License Numbers: 10233 & 10234

Experience the entire NatureBody™ Connection at
www.aquaterramassage.com

Dedicated to your

marvelous,

living,

breathing body.

Index of Reflections

Contents

How to Use This Book

Humans have lived in balance with our bodies and the earth for 2.6 million years. Our bodies are designed for this planet. It is natural to walk on uneven ground, climb mountains, run long distances, swim, and most of all, to deeply breathe fresh air. Our wild planet heals and strengthens us by making us more flexible and fluid.

Your body is born of this earth. Earth is here to support you. Unfortunately, the stresses of life pull us off balance, and can leave us feeling physically sore and mentally anxious. This creative journey into relaxation is a way to remember your natural balance and create new muscle memories.

As massage therapists, we understand how a relaxed body feels: how it breathes, how it moves, how it is balanced in space. This NatureBody™ massage story shares the full spectrum of massage: body, mind and spirit. Our intention is to empower you to find healing within yourself.

Visualization can have powerful effects on your body.[1] In this guided visualization, you will exercise your mind and imagination to deeply relax and bring your body back to center.

If you are injured or your ability to move is limited, then visualization is even more important! Studies have shown that when you imagine moving, the same areas of your brain activate as if you are actually moving those specific muscles.[2] Through visualization, you are virtually exercising your body.

We are intending for you to have a tangible, physical response to the ideas in this book. The power of this story lies in the vividness of your imagination. Read slowly. Pause. Use all of your senses to experience the story. Imagine the changes in humidity. Feel the gentle breeze on your skin. Hear the soothing sound of the wind. Smell the fresh scent of the life around you. Use your vibrant imagination to experience every detail in this story.

Put yourself in the story. Try to experience every sensation in your body. If you feel like moving, do it! Trust your instincts. Imagine what it feels like to move through the story: your muscles warming and stretching... your breathing deepening... your heartbeat slowing as you deeply relax. Let these sensations come to you at the speed of thought. This isn't about concentrating as much as it is about experiencing.

Each time you practice visualizing this story, your experience will become more vibrant. Your body is your wilderness to explore and understand. Your mind is your canvas for new muscle memories.

The Reflections are our personal notes to you. They offer you insight into some of the concepts in the story. Use them to spark your own creative thoughts about connection and healing.

The Notes section is full of wonderful articles and books that we have selected for you. If you feel interested in a topic, we highly recommend you look at the notes to explore the topic further.

The Journal at the end of the book gives you an opportunity to enhance and deepen your meditation. We have asked you a few thought-provoking questions to help you get started. Feel free to write or draw. Journal as creatively as you are inspired. This is your time to dream of the supportive connections between your body and nature.

There is much to discover about your relationship with your body and the beautiful world around you. Find a comfortable place to relax and enjoy. Prepare to be transported to a setting where you can unwind, immersed in nature, and experience the unbridled freedom of the wild!

From Wellness To Oneness,

Erik and Faye
Your Virtual Massage Therapists

FROM WELLNESS TO ONENESS

Wherever you are,

however you feel,

whatever your state of wellness,

know that

healing is at hand.

Your body is always seeking balance

and looking for opportunities to restore.

Through wellness,

may you come to oneness

with your body,

your mind,

your spirit,

and the beautiful Earth that supports us all.

ABOUT THIS MEDITATION

Introduction

We all began our lives floating in our mother's womb. In a sea of amniotic fluid, we took our first strokes to strengthen our newly created bodies.

The ocean holds a special place for us all. Going to the sea is like returning home. When we are gently rocked in the water, we are comforted by the liquid world. Even doing something as simple as taking a bath has a calming influence on our whole being. Our body intuitively remembers our aquatic origins.

Join us in beautiful tropical waters in this NatureBody™ massage story. Let the turquoise waves lull you into serenity. Lie back in the warm, soft sand and savor the sensations of deep relaxation. Relax as you watch palm trees waving in the fresh ocean breeze. Enjoy the expansiveness of the blue sky.

It is thought that life began in the sea. Let us return to the sea to renew our energy and enliven our spirit.

To experience the entire

NatureBody™ Connection

scan this QR code

or go to

www.aquaterramassage.com / naturebodygift / tropicalswim

A gift for you, dear reader.

A special reading by the authors awaits you
at the link above.

CHAPTER ONE

Path to Tranquility

AWAKENING THE SENSES

A narrow path to the beach leads through thick, tropical greenery. Wind-twisted trees arch over the path, their waxy leaves providing deep shade. Flourishing bushes decorated with showy flowers greet me with their tropical aroma.

The path leads to a secluded saltwater lagoon, protected from deep ocean waters by a small coral reef. Palm trees line the beach, lazily reaching toward the lapping water. At the far end of the beach, thickly grown mangroves fill in the spaces between the palms, completing a wave of greenery to the sea.

A tropical breeze floats by. Palm fronds wave gently like long, delicate fingers feeling tendrils of air. A chorus of tropical songbirds sings in the tree canopy, each with its own distinct voice.

Color Healing

"turquoise light...infuses me with the
healing energies of tranquility and renewal."

Color affects your mind and body in subtle ways.[3] The cones in your eyes detect and interpret color, while other receptors send signals to your brain to adjust your body's temperature, blood pressure, mood, and even sleep.[4] Color can increase or suppress your appetite, influence your emotions, and calm or excite your nervous system.[5]

In the morning, when you are surrounded by blue and green light, your brain releases cortisol, which stimulates you to wake up. As that blue-green light darkens into the warm glow of evening, your body releases melatonin to relax and prepare you for sleep.[4]

You can improve your sense of well-being by surrounding yourself with color.

Green and blue are the predominant colors in nature. They have powerful effects on your psychology. Green is both calming and uplifting.[6] Turquoise improves intuition and sensitivity. Seeing the color blue lowers blood pressure, and calms your breathing and heart rate.[7]

Color is a vibration: a wavelength of energy. The vast spectrum of vibrations throughout the planet even radiates colors that the human eye cannot see.[8] Color, and its influence on your body and mood, is a reminder that you are a part of the energy of the universe.

My senses heighten and I feel more alive as I listen to their chirps, whistles, tweets, warbles and trills. The forest behind me teems with bird life. I have this pristine paradise all to myself. I am alone, but not lonely.

Sitting on the warm sand, I stare deeply into the aquamarine water.

My body relaxes in tropical serenity.

Waves lap peacefully on the shore. Crystal clear water sparkles in the gentle sunlight. I see through the shallows to the sand below.

My eyes are bathed in turquoise light.
This color infuses me with the healing energies
of tranquility and renewal.

Sunlight gently illuminates the sand. Shadows of palm trees wave on the shoreline.

My feet sink into the warm, soft sand.
A light breeze spirals around my legs.

The sweet, delicate fragrance of flowers
mingles with the salty sea air.

Sun warms my back and shoulders.
I can feel them melting,
surrendering to gravity.

The tropical breeze cools the heat of my skin.
My neck lengthens.
I feel deeply warm.

CHAPTER TWO

Communing with the Sea

CIRCULATION AND UNDERWATER MASSAGE

The blue-green water complements the azure sky. I am embraced in a world of turquoise: the color of intuition and clarity and calm. A trickle of perspiration travels down my neck. It is time to cool down.

The cool water looks inviting. I walk down the warm sand to the water's edge. Waves lap up the beach and tickle my toes. The water is cool and refreshing.

> Water wraps around my ankles, cooling my feet
> and sending an invigorating rush up to my core.

> I bury my toes in the watery sand,
> spreading them wide to feel the sand
> slide between them.

The Power of Cool Water

> *"My warm skin tingles as the cool water*
> *rises over the backs of my knees."*

Humans have been using the thermal properties of water therapeutically for thousands of years.[9] Cold water has many healing benefits. It stimulates our circulation, eases depression, and decreases tension and fatigue.[10]

Our bodies respond positively to cold temperatures. When we immerse ourselves in cold water, the stress on our bodies stimulates our fight-or-flight response. This elevates the amount of dopamine and norepinephrine in our brains, easing depression, and leaving us with a feeling of being uplifted and energized. The stimulation of our nervous system also increases our metabolism and boosts our immunity.

When you get very hot, you can cool yourself by applying cold compresses. Applying cool to the places where veins run close to your skin, is particularly effective. The inside of your wrists, your elbows, the backs of your knees, between your legs, or under your arms[11] are effective places to cool a warm body.

Our muscles and tissues love movement and flow. Cold water stimulates our circulation by constricting our blood vessels, pushing fluid out of the cooled area. Our warm-blooded bodies naturally reheat, dilating our blood vessels. This sends a rush of fresh, nutrient-rich fluid into the area. By alternating between hot and cold temperatures, you invite circulation to your tissues. Cool water is a powerful tool to heal your body.

I walk out into the water, and feel the gentle press of the sea. In this protected lagoon, there are no crashing waves, but only gentle swells.

The cool water feels wonderful
on my deeply warmed skin.

My legs relish the contrast.

My warm skin tingles
as the cool water rises over the backs of my knees.

I stand here,
feeling the swaying
push and pull
of the surf on my legs.

I bend my knees, throw my hands up over my head and dive out into the water!

My whole body tenses for a split second
and then expands into relief.

Circulation surges through me
as my capillaries constrict in the cool water.

The experience is energizing!

Eager to explore the lagoon, I swim the crystal clear shallows out to the life-giving coral reef. Seagrass sways back and forth in the rhythmic pulsing of the water. A turtle swims below me, its front flippers waving as it propels herself gracefully forward. The turtle's shadow undulates on the rippling sand below.

Rocking Yourself to Health

"The underwater world seems to be undulating, rocking peacefully in rhythm to the heartbeat of the ocean."

The motion of rocking is very soothing. Just as rocking a baby lulls them to sleep, rocking has a profoundly relaxing effect on our adult bodies throughout our lives.

Our affinity for rocking began in utero. Our mother's movements created a fluid, rocking motion in the womb. This rhythmic motion stimulated our brain, giving us tremendous amounts of sensory information, such as where our heads and necks were positioned in space as we moved.[12]

As infants, rocking continued to develop our vestibular system: the system that helps us balance, track moving objects, and learn fine motor skills.[13]

As adults, being rocked helps you go to sleep faster, and enter a dream state more quickly. Whether you rock in a hammock or rocking chair, or go for a ride in a car or train, the feeling of your body moving can help you sleep more deeply.[14] The soothing act of rocking influences the wavelengths of your mind. Being gently rocked while you sleep synchronizes the brainwaves that help improve your memory.[15]

Rocking nurtures your brain and comforts your body. Who would have thought a little time in a rocking chair or swinging in a hammock could be so valuable?

There is an abundance of sea life below the tranquil waves. A clownfish swims through the gentle fingers of a sea anemone. Small sea fan corals wave slowly back and forth, visually affirming the rhythm of the ocean. A school of little yellow fish swims by, their scales glinting in the diffuse sunlight. I watch them move effortlessly with little sideways flicks of their tails.

The underwater world seems to be undulating, rocking peacefully in harmony with the heartbeat of the ocean. My body floats easily in the salt water.

I feel at home in this lagoon.

My hair floats around me
    and my fingers relax and spread
    in this floating world.

My body blends
    into the peaceful swaying of the sea.

I let my legs go,
    feeling them naturally relax
    into their most comfortable position.

The full body peace envelops me.

I feel each muscle release.

My spine floats freely,
    the discs becoming more fluid.

Exhaling to Breathe

*"I exhale and watch bubbles rise up to the surface,
each one glinting in the sun like crystal."*

The key to a full, satisfying breath lies in the exhale. Exhaling fully empties your lungs of stale air. Your next inhale naturally feels more satisfying.

Many of us overemphasize our inhales, trying to take fuller and fuller breaths. We tense our necks and chest muscles to inflate our lungs. It is almost as though we are gasping for air. Breathing this way is not only inefficient, but it also tenses our muscles and stresses our nervous system.

A full exhale leaves your lungs more available for a satisfying inhale. When you exhale completely, you no longer need to over-inflate your lungs to get a satisfying breath. A regular inhale is enough to replenish your oxygen. Your nervous system calms and your muscles can relax.[16]

On your next breath, fully exhale all the air out of your lungs. Squeeze your air out completely. Cough the last bit of air out. Hold your breath out for a count of four, then allow your next inhale to fill you. You do not need to inhale deeply: just let it come naturally. When you are ready, exhale fully again. For an added challenge, try breathing in and out through your nose, which enhances the replenishing sensation of breathing.

Full exhales are the starting point for finding a deeply refreshing, ultra relaxing, and satisfying breath.

The light is complex and deep.

As the water ripples,
    dappled light swirls and moves,
    marbling the seascape like a living silk painting.

I dive down to touch the painting.

The penetrating light
    gives the ocean a gothic radiance.

The ripples are soft down here,
    the sun's gleaming rays
    dancing through them.

I exhale
    and watch bubbles rise to the surface,
    each one glinting in the sun like crystal.

Following the bubbles up,
    their lens-like shapes grow
    as they rise
    through the liquid atmosphere.

When I emerge from the aquatic realm,
    I take a large, refreshing breath of air.

I feel renewed and relaxed
    as I lie back in the water
    and float on its surface.

CHAPTER THREE

Floating on the Surface

FREEDOM OF THE SPINE AND CHEST MASSAGE

Saltwater buoys me as I float. I arch my back and kick lightly, gazing up at the puffy white clouds. Water ripples around my face and chest.

> *My head rests back in the water,*
> *which submerges my ears.*

> *I listen to the sounds of the underwater world.*

> *I am at once a part of the watery world below*
> *and the heavenly world above.*

A frigate bird flies overhead with its signature split tail. It soars in the breeze above as I float in the water, rocked by the gentle waves. I watch the bird until it disappears in the distance.

Opening Your Chest

*"I pull my shoulders back into the water,
arching my back as my chest continues to widen."*

Swimming is a fantastic activity that tones your whole bodies and encourages you to move in new ways. Floating and doing the backstroke help stretch your chest and rebalance your posture.[7]

On land, our activities tend to round our shoulders forward. Whether we are driving, reading, working at the computer, or cooking, when our hands are in front of us, our chest muscles shorten, which pulls our shoulders forward. The muscles between our shoulder blades become overstretched and ropey, and blood does not flow through them as well.

The backstroke moves your shoulders through their whole range of motion. Stretch your arms up above your head, and strongly reach around and behind you. These large motions stretch your chest muscles and encourage your shoulder blades onto their balanced home on your back.

To find this feeling on land, use light weights or resistance bands to mimic the resistance of water. Spread your arms wide to open your chest and squeeze your shoulder blades together. As you strengthen your back muscles and stretch your chest muscles, your posture improves.

The mild resistance of water is a great way to explore your joint health and tone your body. Enjoy your next swim!

My arms spread wide,
    opening my shoulders and upper body.

I pull my shoulders back into the water,
    arching my back as my chest continues to widen.

I breathe in fully to remain buoyant.

My expanded chest breaks the surface,
    bathed in the warm tropical sun.

My neck lengthens as I present myself to the sky.

I feel my scalp sliding back
    as I open my face to the radiant light above.

My legs drop and my hips open,
    completing my body's long arch.

I am enjoying the contrasting sensations
    of warm sunlight on my chest
    and the cool swirls of water that float over my torso.

When I move my arms, water ripples between my fingers.

Bobbing up and down with the water,
    my neck relaxes and releases.

My body undulates with
    the small ripples and surges of the sea.

I am connected to the living ocean.

CHAPTER FOUR

Swimming Back to Shore

SHOULDER, HIP, AND LEG MASSAGE

I roll over and begin to swim slowly back to shore. My legs kick alternately and my hips open, each hemisphere of my pelvis moving independently. My leg and its associated hip feel like they are connected, front, back, inside and outside.

My legs act as extensions of my dynamic pelvis. I offset the motion of my kick with my strong core. My legs extend and reach, working in alternating rhythm.

I am recruiting many of my muscles to swim. Even kicking my legs becomes a supported, full body effort. All of my movements radiate out from my core, as if the goal were to carry my navel home.

The delightful sensations of movement travel through me.

The Action of Thought

"My rehearsed movements become more natural."

All movements begin in the mind. Before your muscles actually fire, your brain instructs your body how to move.[18] Every movement is first completed mentally. Then your body performs.

Visualizing your movements can help you move more efficiently. From top athletes[19] to people rehabilitating from medical setbacks,[20] visualization has been shown to be a powerful tool in improving performance. Visualizing an activity stimulates your brain in the same ways as actually performing that activity.[21] In fact, research has shown that visualizing heavy lifting can actually make your muscles stronger![22] Your mind is powerful. It can help set you on the right path.

Mentally rehearse your movements. Visualize yourself doing every aspect of the movement, from preparation to cooling down. Picture every sensation as you visualize yourself moving. Use as many senses as you can to animate your thoughts. What do you see, hear, feel, smell and taste as you move? Let your imagination bring you into the moment.

Your mind sets the pace for your body to follow.

It all starts with a thought.

I feel the tone of my muscles
  drawing me tighter to my core
  while my fingers and toes
  reach farther away.

My bones remain comfortably saddled in their joints
  as my muscles move long and freely.

I reach forward and press the water back.

My shoulder moves fully,
  from fully lengthened
  to fully contracted.

I imagine my pinky finger reaching tall
  all the way from my pinky toe.

As I extend each arm up overhead,
  my ribcage stretches,
  further expanding my reach.

Bringing my arms down to my sides,
  I experience the contraction of my side body.

This rhythmic pumping of muscles
  brings nourishing circulation to their tissues.

I focus deeper on each motion. My rehearsed movements
become more natural. My mind is free to dream.

The Graceful Sea Lion

*"I pretend I am a sea lion. I move gracefully
through this turquoise world."*

Sea lions emerge from the water and lumber up on land, awkwardly flopping their bodies around to find a perfect place to warm in the sun. Their bodies are not designed to move well on land. Underwater, however, they move as gracefully as ballet dancers. Sea lions are sleek and elegant underwater. The sea is their home. In the water, they twist and turn, glide and curl in a beautiful dance, spiraling their bodies around effortlessly.

Like a sea lion, there are movements you do that feel perfectly natural, and others that are awkward and difficult. When you are learning something new, begin by moving in ways that you have learned in the past. Then modify your movements to adapt to the new activity. Your old muscle memories provide a foundation for you to learn new activities, and create new muscle memories.

Training in water can be a powerful aid to help you learn more strenuous activities. Rehearse new movements in a pool. The lack of gravity and the added resistance of water help you build strength without impact on your joints. There is even a form of massage that takes place in water. Watsu® is a shiatsu massage where you float in warm water and are passively moved and stretched by a massage therapist.

Be patient with yourself as you learn new activities. Grace comes with practice.

As I continue back to the beach, I dive down underwater.

I propel myself forward,
    my spine undulating in fluid rhythm.

I pretend I am a sea lion.
    I move gracefully
    through this turquoise world.

My spine opens with its wavelike movement,
    lengthening and loosening
    the soft discs between the bones.

I swim past a vibrant patch of sea grass, its luminescent green contrasting with the pale white sand.

I wave my hand above the grass
    to watch its green leaves wave back at me.

I surface again and swim lazily back to shore. The water warms as I near the beach.

I revel in the refreshing warmth of this perfect tropical bath.

I swim until my belly touches the sand, and I rise heavily from all fours to standing.

CHAPTER FIVE

Unwinding on the Beach

FULL BODY RELAXATION

Gravity, the cohesive force that all mass is subject to, and holds our planet together, weighs heavily on me now as I emerge from the water and walk across the beach. My body feels wonderfully worked and refreshed from my swim.

The beach is lovely, lightly shaded by palm trees. My feet make deep prints in the warm, pillowy sand.

I lie down under a palm tree, letting the sun's warmth penetrate my belly, chest and legs. Gravity feels heavy and comforting.

> *My body sinks into the warm sand,*
> *allowing my muscles to relax.*

On Sun and Gravity

*"My body deepens its relaxation as I invite this energy
into every tissue from head to fingers, legs to toes."*

One great technique to relaxing is to do an enhanced body scan. Get comfortable. Lie back with your head supported. Focus on each area of your body from head to toe.

A body scan is a meditation that can help you feel more connected to your body. It can help relieve chronic pain[23] and bring you into the rest-and-relax nervous mode.

Heat brings circulation to your body: a feeling of flow and life force. Gravity is a dependable force that can be used to encourage your muscles to unwind and relax.

Begin by focusing on your head. Breathe. Imagine the heat of the sun deeply warming your whole head. As you inhale, become aware of the sensations within your head. What do you feel? Exhale, and let your head sink back with the weight gravity.

Continue scanning, one body part at a time, from head to toe, until your whole body is relaxed.

Warm your tissues.
Inhale awareness.
Exhale into heaviness.
"Warm. Breathe. Release."

Visualize yourself melting into the earth. Feel your body blending into and becoming one with the planet.

I keep my eyes closed
as I soak in the golden heat of the sun.

Warmth penetrates my chest and abdomen,
allowing a feeling of deep relaxation
to envelop my body.

I allow my sternum to widen
and my shoulders to sink to the sand.

My jaw relaxes.
My throat softens.

My chin sinks down toward my throat,
while the top of my head reaches,
lengthening my neck.

As the sun warms me,
I feel its healing energy
radiate deeply through me.

My body deepens its relaxation
as I invite this energy into every tissue
from head to fingers,
legs to toes.

A light breeze washes over me,
contrasting exquisitely to the deep warmth within.

The gentle lapping of the waves on the shore and the rustling of the palms in the breeze, soothe me into tranquility.

CHAPTER SIX

Gratitude

A BLESSING FROM THE SEA

T hank you for joining me at this beautiful beach today. Until we meet again,

> May you breathe deeply,
>   as if you have just emerged from the sea.
>
> May the dance of the ocean buoy you
>   when gravity gets you down.
>
> May the heat of the sun renew
>   the waves of circulation in your tissues.
>
> May the sands of time remind you
>   of the peace of this moment.
>
> May your life be as creative, joyful, and full of possibility,
>   as all of the colorful fish in the sea.

Float on, Tranquil Wanderer. May our paths merge again.

Acknowledgments

My first scuba diving trip sparked a lifelong interest in our oceans. Many thanks to my uncle, Bill Bollinger, for being a fun and adventurous diving partner. Taking my first deep dive, orienteering underwater at night, and exploring shipwrecks made our adventure profoundly memorable.

I am deeply grateful to my grandparents, Edith and Ralph Bollinger. After being married in New Caledonia while serving in the military during World War II, their love of the South Pacific was forever present in their lives. You encouraged me to dream bigger, adventure farther, and to hold the warm spirit of being in service to another in my heart.

Thank you to the crew of the sailing vessel, *Tui Tai*. You introduced us to a truly beautiful experience with lifelong memories. It was delightful to sail, play, snorkel and swim in the warm tropical waters of the South Pacific. Being embraced by the warmth and generosity of the Fijian people touched us. We were fascinated with their deep connection to nature: to learn of the constellations, the medicinal plants, and the traditional customs on these remote islands in the South Pacific.

We deeply appreciate Sylvia Earle's lifelong work of caring for the oceans. We thoroughly enjoyed her documentary, *Mission Blue*.

James Cameron's spirit of exploration brought him to the deepest oceans with his submarine, the Deepsea Challenger. He inspired the world to care for places yet unexplored.

BBC Earth's documentary, *Blue Planet*, inspired us with their beautiful depiction of the various splendors of the seas.

The BBC series, *Nature's Most Amazing Events* shows how the flow of water throughout the planet influences all life. The episode, *The Great Feast*, showed how humpback whales give birth and raise their young in the safety of warm tropical waters.

Notes

1. "What is Imagery?" *Johns Hopkins Medicine*, 2003, www.hopkinsmedicine.org/health/wellness-and-prevention/imagery.

2. Lohr, Jim. "Can Visualizing Your Body Doing Something Help You Learn to Do It Better?" *Scientific American*, 1 May 2015, www.scientificamerican.com/article/can-visualizing-your-body-doing-something-help-you-learn-to-do-it-better.

3. Nicola, Stephanie. "What is Color Psychology? *WebMD*, 27 April 2022, www.webmd.com/mental-health/what-is-color-psychology.

4. Westland, Stephen. "Here's How Colours Really Affect Our Brain And Body, According to Science." *ScienceAlert*, 28 September 2017, www.sciencealert.com/does-colour-really-affect-our-brain-and-body-a-professor-of-colour-science-explains.

5. Cherry, Kendra. "Color Psychology: Does It Affect How You Feel?" *Very Well Mind,* 9 November 2022, www.verywellmind.com/color-psychology-2795824.

6. Pichardo, Gabriela. "How Colors Can Affect You." *WebMD,* 5 September 2021, www.webmd.com/balance/ss/slideshow-colors-affect-you.

7. Al-Ayash, Aseel & Kane, Robert & Smith, Dianne & Green-Armytage, Paul. "The Influence of Color on Student Emotion, Heart Rate, and Performance in Learning Environments." *ResearchGate,* April 2016, www.researchgate.net/publication/340739120_The_Influence_of_Color_on_Student_Emotion_Heart_Rate_and_Performance_in_Learning_Environments.

8. Hathaway-Yale, Bill. "Birds See Colors Invisible To Humans." *Futurity,* 23 June 2011, www.futurity.org/birds-see-colors-invisible-to-humans.

9. Marchetti, Sylvia. "Archaeologists Recover Ancient 'Fertility Statuettes' From Famed Tuscan Hot Springs." *CNN,* 10 August 2022, www.cnn.com/style/article/san-casciano-dei-bagni-thermal-baths-relics-scn/index.html.

10. Stanborough, Rebecca Joy. "What to Know About Cold Water Therapy." *Healthline,* 8 July 2020, www.healthline.com/health/cold-water-therapy.

11. Gordon, Whitson. "Know Your Body's Quick-Cooling Spots." *Lifehacker,* 25 June 2010, lifehacker.com/know-your-bodys-quick-cooling-spots-5571072.

12. "What Is the Vestibular Sense & Why Is It Important For Child Development?" *Children Inspired By Yoga,* childreninspiredbyyoga.com/blog/2018/01/vestibular-sense-child-development. Accessed on 30 January 2023.

13. Sandler, A., & Coren, A. "Vestibular Stimulation in Early Childhood: A Review." *Journal of the Division for Early Childhood*, vol. 3, no. 1, 1981, pp. 48–55, doi.org/10.1177/105381518100300108.

14. "Swaying of Hammock Lulls Brain into Deeper Sleep." *NPR*, 24 June 2011, www.npr.org/2011/06/24/137397961/swaying-of-hammock-lulls-brain-into-deeper-sleep.

15. Sandoiu, Ana. "Why Being Rocked Will Help You Sleep Better." *Medical News Today*, 25 January 2019, www.medicalnewstoday.com/articles/324275.

16. Polatin, Betsy. "Breath in Motion: Why Exhaling Matters Most." *Huffington Post*, 21 February 2014, www.huffpost.com/entry/breath-in-motionwhy-exhal_b_4769819.

17. "4 Different Swimming Strokes and Their Benefits." *CureJoy*, 8 October 2019, curejoy.com/content/different-swimming-strokes-and-their-benefits.

18. "Left or Right? The Brain Knows Before You Move." *Howard Hughes Medical Institute*, 26 February 2015, www.hhmi.org/news/left-or-right-brain-knows-you-move.

19. Quinn, Elizabeth. "How Imagery and Visualization Can Improve Athletic Performance." *Very Well Fit*, 4 July 2021, www.verywellfit.com/visualization-techniques-for-athletes-3119438.

20. "Mental Practice for Stroke Patients: How to Use Visualization to Boost Your Recovery." *Flint Rehab*, 6 October 2022, www.flintrehab.com/mental-practice-stroke-rehabilitation.

21. Schnitzler A, Salenius S, Salmelin R, Jousmäki V, Hari R. "Involvement of Primary Motor Cortex in Motor Imagery: A Neuromagnetic Study." *Neuroimage*, vol. 6, no. 3, 1997, pp. 201-208, doi:10.1006/nimg.1997.0286.

22. Ranganathan, V. K., Siemionow, V., Liu, J. Z., Sahgal, V., & Yue, G. H. "From Mental Power to Muscle Power-Gaining Strength by Using the Mind." *Neuropsychologia*, vol. 42 no. 7, 2004, pp. 944–956. doi.org/10.1016/j.neuropsychologia.2003.11.018.

23. Mccubbin, Tracy et al. "Mindfulness-based stress reduction in an integrated care delivery system: one-year impacts on patient-centered outcomes and health care utilization." *The Permanente Journal*, vol. 18, no. 4, 2014, pp. 4-9. doi:10.7812/TPP/14-014.

MEDITATION

Journal

This journal gives you a place to reflect on your experience as you read and meditate. With every meditation, your library of personal affirmations can grow. Some thoughts you might want to record, in words or drawings, are:

Describe the tropical beach paradise you envision. Write about your vision of yourself on your beach: physically, mentally and emotionally.

Notice and describe how you react to different colors. Which colors do you think of when you relax?

What creatures of the sea would you enjoy moving like? Swimming like a sea lion? Stretching like a starfish? Crawling like a crab? Swaying like sea grass?

How does rocking make you feel?

Enjoy dreaming of your body in nature, and exploring the nature of your body.

"I STAND HERE, FEELING THE
SWAYING PUSH AND PULL
OF THE SURF ON MY LEGS."

MEDITATION

You are deeply connected to the energy of the outside world. Within your body and throughout Earth, natural forces rhythmically ebb and flow. The circulation inside you and the thrum of your heartbeat resonates with the lunar tides and currents of the ocean. The push and the pull of outside forces can influence your balance, your emotions, and your thoughts, but they need not pull you off center. In the constantly shifting energies of the world, you remain standing. You are intimately joined with the great sea.

~

"I AM ALONE, BUT NOT LONELY. I
HAVE THIS PRISTINE PARADISE
ALL TO MYSELF."

MEDITATION

In nature, you are never truly alone: you are encircled by the living beings of the planet: the trees, the moss, the animals, birds and insects. When you feel alone, close your eyes and listen: you will begin to notice the subtle sounds of life all around you. You are not a singularity: you are intimately connected to this living world.

~

May you

BREATHE

DEEPLY

as if you just

emerged

from the sea.

"THE UNDERWATER WORLD SEEMS
TO BE UNDULATING, ROCKING
PEACEFULLY IN HARMONY WITH
THE HEARTBEAT OF THE OCEAN."

MEDITATION

The underwater world is tangibly and viscously connected to the rhythms of Earth. Our lives up on the surface feel more airy and free, but the connection runs as deep. We are always being held and supported by the creative forces that made us.

Picture yourself held and supported by the creative forces of Earth. Imagine the connection between you and Earth so vividly that your living energy feels as thickly viscous as the sea. As you feel this connection within, you enrich your relationship with that which has created you.

~

"MY FEET SINK INTO THE SOFT, WARM SAND. A LIGHT BREEZE SPIRALS AROUND MY LEGS."

MEDITATION

Imagine yourself standing on a sandy beach. The sand is soft and warm. As your feet sink into the sand, picture your toes spreading as sand fills the spaces between them. Visualize your energy projecting down deep into the Earth. You are energetically connecting to all that is.

~

May the

DANCE

of the

OCEAN

buoy you

when gravity

gets you down.

"I AM ENJOYING THE CONTRASTING
SENSATIONS OF WARM SUNLIGHT
ON MY CHEST AND THE COOL
SWIRLS OF WATER THAT FLOAT
OVER MY TORSO."

MEDITATION

Your body is continually stimulated by outside sensation: hot and cold, soft and rough, dry and wet. These tactile sensations awaken your senses to the world around you.

There are times when these sensations go unnoticed: where you are focused elsewhere and do not notice the stimuli you are experiencing. At other times, a single drop of water, or slight feeling of chill, can bring a world of sensation.

Through different valences of consciousness, you sensitize yourself to the world around you. Sometimes, it is necessary to desensitize yourself in order to make forward progress. Other times, it is important to feel the nuances and allow yourself to become deeply aware of what your body is experiencing: to listen as your body speaks to you.

~

"I ARCH MY BACK AND KICK
LIGHTLY, GAZING UP AT THE
CLOUDS AND LISTENING TO THE
WATER RIPPLE AROUND ME."

MEDITATION

Floating gives us the feeling of being buoyed and supported by water. It takes practice to float comfortably: to develop the skill to relax your body into the support of water. Being able to let go of the physical mechanics required to float allows you to become aware in the moment. You become conscious of the sounds of water next to your ears, and have the presence to behold the sky and look beyond to the heavens above.

~

May the

HEAT

of the

SUN

renew

the waves of circulation

in your tissues.

"ALL OF MY MOVEMENTS RADIATE
OUT FROM MY CORE, AS IF THE
GOAL WERE TO CARRY MY NAVEL
HOME."

MEDITATION

Your center of gravity contains the source that allows for healthy and balanced expansion. A strong abdominal core gives you the support you need to reach and stretch farther.

In life, when you have a strong core of supportive family and friends, you feel more free to shine: to let your unique energy radiate out to the world.

~

.   .   .   .

.   .   .   .

.   .   .   .

.   .   .   .

.   .   .   .

"MY EYES ARE BATHED IN
TURQUOISE LIGHT. THIS COLOR
INFUSES MY BODY WITH THE
HEALING ENERGIES OF
TRANQUILITY AND RENEWAL."

.   .   .   .

.   .   .   .

.   .   .   .

.   .   .   .

.   .   .   .

.   .   .   .

MEDITATION

What colors do you see when you look around? The colors your eyes detect influence the way you feel and see the world.

Imagine you are in a forest. See the varieties of greens and browns all around you.

Imagine you are in an arid desert. Yellows and oranges in the landscape contrast with a rich blue sky.

Imagine you are at the ocean, surrounded by blues of every shade.

How do you feel as you picture each of these settings? Can you feel yourself respond to the colors?

~

May the

SANDS

of

TIME

remind you

of the peace

of this moment.

"I FOCUS DEEPER ON EACH MOTION.
MY REHEARSED MOVEMENTS
BECOME MORE NATURAL. MY MIND
IS FREE TO DREAM."

MEDITATION

Your body has evolved in the natural world and instinctively understands how to move. Becoming naturally adept at new activities can take a lot of effort and rehearsal. Through practice, the mental theory of new movement evolves into a full body knowing. As you practice, you become more natural: your body flows effortlessly, and you can be present in your awareness of the world around you. You have become a master.

There is a time when the student stops studying and naturally takes their knowledge out into the world, to give to others.

~

"THE GENTLE LAPPING OF
THE WAVES ON THE SHORE, AND
THE RUSTLING OF THE PALMS IN
THE BREEZE, SOOTHES ME INTO
DEEP RELAXATION."

MEDITATION

When you are in nature, your body responds to the vibrations around you...

...the song of crickets in the evening.
...the crashing waves on the shore.
...the steady push of the breeze through the trees.

These natural sounds soothe our bodies on a deep level: like the comforting sensation of being gently rocked into relaxation.

What sounds do you hear?

~

May your

LIFE

be as

CREATIVE,

JOYFUL,

and

FULL OF POSSIBILITY

as all

of the colorful

fish in the sea.

> "SUN WARMS MY BACK AND
> SHOULDERS. I CAN FEEL THEM
> RELAXING WITH GRAVITY,
> BECOMING BROADER
> WITH EACH BREATH."

MEDITATION

As our tissues heat up, they become more pliable. Our warmed, relaxed bodies can move more fluidly.

When we become tense, the pressures of life can feel like they are squeezing in on us. It is as if we become smaller. Our body contracts inward and our breathing becomes more shallow.

To breathe deeply into your warm, relaxed body is to expand into the natural space your body was born to inhabit.

~

"AS THE SUN WARMS ME,
I FEEL ITS HEALING ENERGY
RADIATE DEEPLY THROUGH ME."

MEDITATION

Imagine how you feel on a summer day, when the sun's warmth penetrates your muscles and bones. Feel your body soften and relax as you accept the deep heat. The sun's warmth energizes you to the core. Your thoughts float away, and your body vibrates with living energy. A sense of calm washes over you.

As you tune in to the stimuli around you, you can focus these feelings to give your body a sense of relaxation and your mind a feeling of freedom. The sensations of the natural world can enhance your feeling of being embraced in belonging.

~

BLESSING
FROM THE SEA

May you
BREATHE DEEPLY
as if you have just emerged from the sea.

May the
DANCE OF THE OCEAN
buoy you when gravity gets you down.

May the
HEAT OF THE SUN
renew the waves of circulation in your tissues.

May the
SANDS OF TIME
remind you of the peace of this moment.

May your
LIFE
be as
CREATIVE,
JOYFUL,
and
FULL OF POSSIBILITY
as all of the colorful fish in the sea.

About the Authors

Born and raised in New Orleans, Erik Krippner grew up with a po'boy in his hand and a song in his heart. As a boy, he spent his summers swimming, hiking, fishing, and sailing. After becoming an Eagle Scout, Erik dreamed of answering the call to "Go West, young man." He earned a Bachelor of Science degree in Forestry from Louisiana State University. Following his passion for adventure, Erik found his way to the mountains of the Pacific Northwest, his home to this day. After working in the forests of Oregon, Washington, Idaho, Alaska, Georgia, and Louisiana, Erik decided to focus his love of natural sciences on the study of human body through massage therapy.

Faye grew up in Oregon surrounded by family and old growth coastal forests. She spent many childhood weekends cross-country skiing, hunting for mushrooms, exploring coastal tide pools, and searching for crawdads in the Siuslaw River. Her love of books deepened when she became the editor of her high school and college's literary journals. Upon earning her Bachelor of Arts degree in Mathematics with honors from the Robert D. Clark Honors College at the University of Oregon, Faye became a technical writer and web developer. The whisper of a deeper purpose ignited her to study massage, where she met Erik.

Erik and Faye became friends in massage school at the East West College of the Healing Arts, in Portland, Oregon. In 2003, they founded Aqua Terra Massage, a therapeutic massage studio for friends and couples. Since then, they have practiced therapeutic massage together, side by side. They have spent years immersed in the study of massage, serving thousands of clients.

Faye and Erik have spent years exploring and writing about our beautiful world. They have sailed the blue waters of Fiji's Koro Sea, kayaked New Zealand's Marlborough Sound, and stargazed among the giraffes and elephants in Botswana. They have hiked the Appalachian Trail and paddled the tidally-influenced Columbia River in the Pacific Northwest. They have seen orca whales swim right under their kayaks, locked eyes with wild lions, and played hide-and-seek with an octopus. They have hiked thousands of miles together, kayaked and sailed hundreds, and spent countless evenings camping under the stars.

With a commitment to bringing more love and kindness
to this beautiful world, we offer this book to you.

www.aquaterramassage.com

Made in the USA
Monee, IL
29 May 2023

34270272R00059